Water Fasting & Dry Fasting for Beginners

Merryl Kowalska

Published by Merryl Kowalska, 2023.

While every precaution has been taken in the preparation of this book, the publisher assumes no responsibility for errors or omissions, or for damages resulting from the use of the information contained herein.

WATER FASTING & DRY FASTING FOR BEGINNERS

First edition. January 10, 2023.

Copyright © 2023 Merryl Kowalska.

ISBN: 979-8215651292

Written by Merryl Kowalska.

Also by Merryl Kowalska

Immersive Magic
A Guide to Acquiring an Astral Magic Wand
Solitary Witchcraft for Beginners
Faerie Magick for Beginners
Magical Experiments That You Can Do at Home
Pendulum Dowsing Mastery Codex
White Magic Manual
Immersive Magic: Creating Energy Constructs
Beat Casino Games Using Psychic Techniques

Standalone
How to Be a Freelance Writer
Conjuration of the Demon Eryezel
Magical Cleansing and Defensive Techniques
Magick Black Book: Creating Magical Imbalances
The I Am of All Things and the None Self
Water Fasting & Dry Fasting for Beginners

Watch for more at https://www.czlibrary.com/.

Table of Contents

For Janne

Introduction

Water Fasting & Dry Fasting for Beginners is a life manual that teaches the ancient healing and spiritual art of water fasting, as well as dry fasting. Fasting has been used for centuries as a powerful tool for healing and spiritual growth. What is water fasting? Water fasting is abstaining from food for a certain period of time. It is a time where you can only consume pure and clean water, and nothing more. Dry fasting takes it a step further where you do not consume any food and water for a period of time.

If you are just starting out, water fasting is the way to go. Once you gain more experience and confidence, you can easily shift from water fasting into a pure dry fasting. Nevertheless, it should be noted that there are many spiritual seekers and even health enthusiasts who are already satisfied with water fasting and have no interest in doing a dry fast. You can also do the same, if you want. Feel free to do whatever makes you feel good, clean, and healthy.

Water Fasting & Dry Fasting for Beginners teaches the ins and outs of fasting. Fasting is not a new invention. It has been in existence since ancient times for various purposes, mainly for religious, spiritual, and health purposes. I have practiced both water and dry fasting for years, and I am here to share with you everything that I have learned.

Before we move further, I want you to know that water fasting (as well as dry fasting) is very much doable. You just have to give yourself enough time to adjust.

If you want to be healthy and enjoy a deeper experience of spirituality, then water/dry fasting might just be the way to satisfy your spiritual cravings. This practice is deeply experiential, and it can even change you as a person. In fact, many of those who seriously go on a fast experience a wonderful and pleasant state of mind, and such a state of mind can only be achieved through the practice of fasting.

Although there are many ways to do fasting, it remains true that there are really only two original ways of fasting, and that is through a water fast or a dry fast. As far as this book is concerned, we shall use the term *fast* or *fasting* to refer to both water and dry fasting, except when clearly specified to mean otherwise.

So, are you ready to learn the wonders of fasting? If yes, then without further ado, let us begin your journey to health, peace of mind, well-being, and spirituality.

On Fasting

Fasting is one of the best and ancient ways to good health and spirituality. In our modern world, we are often bombarded with so many things to consume. Sadly, many of the foods and drinks that we have are bad for our health. In fact, they are so bad that people are getting sick from them. Of course, the modern world would not want you to know about all this to ensure the continuous flow of profits, at your expense.

Many of the world's greatest people have also engaged in fasting. An excellent example of this would be Jesus, Buddha, and Moses, among so many others. Pythagoras also practiced fasting. In fact, fasting was a part of the requirements before Pythagoras would take anyone in as a disciple.

But why would anyone go on a fast? What can fasting do for you?

Fasting has many benefits. For starters, fasting will allow you to take control of the flesh, as well as the desires of the flesh. By learning to control your appetite, you can easily take control of other worldly desires. If you want to develop more discipline and self-control, then fasting would be very helpful.

If you feel like your mind is always bombarded with so many negative thoughts and the ceaseless stuff of the modern world, fasting can help you heal your mind and soul. Fasting is known for helping one achieve a clear and deep state of mind and being.

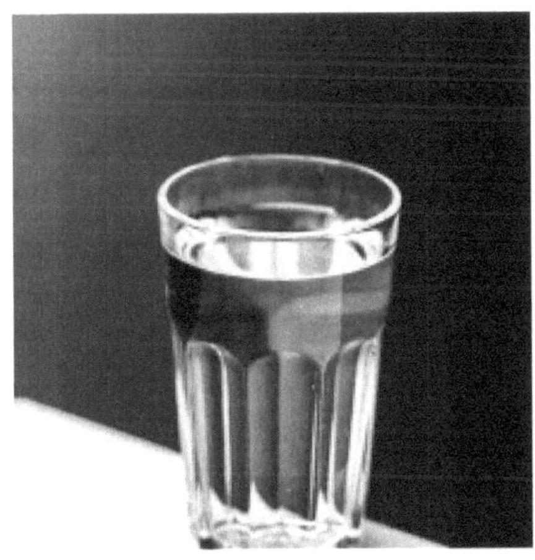

Fasting was also used in the mystical schools in ancient Greece and Egypt. Before initiates of the sacred knowledge would be handed new teachings, they would be required to fast in order to prepare their mind to receive the teachings.

With regard to the physical health benefits of fasting, this is something that conventional science has also proven to be effective. Fasting is a very powerful way to heal. It should be noted that the physical body is designed as a powerful healing machine. However, in our modern world, the body is often bombarded with so many unhealthy foods and drinks to digest, which cripples the body's innate healing power. When you go on a fast, you will be able to activate the full healing potential of the human body, which would have the way to healing various diseases and sicknesses.

Fasting has also been practiced by various monks from different traditions, as well as by so many spiritual seekers. If you want to get more in touch with your soul, then fasting is the way to go.

Many times, we become too attached to our physical body that we forget the most basic universal principle that we are, first and foremost, a soul. The physical body is yours, but it is not you. By becoming more connected to the soul, you can discover who you really are and what really matters most in your life instead of wasting your life with meaningless and shallow things.

Fasting is also a proven way to strengthen one's aura. The aura is an energy field that surrounds the body. A strong aura reflects a healthy mind and body. By strengthening your aura, you will also enjoy peace of mind and a stronger body.

If losing weight is your objective, then fasting is a very effective way to lose weight. There are those who say that you will only be losing water weight when you fast; but based on my personal experience, this is really not the case. Indeed, you will also be losing water weight, but you will also lose those stubborn fats and burn those calories. In fact, based on my experience, I was able to lose more weight going on a water fast (and sometimes a dry fast) than doing a keto diet with daily one-hour exercise.

There are many other benefits of fasting. Nevertheless, the best and only way to experience and actually enjoy them is through actual and personal experience.

Is It for Me?

A common misconception about fasting is that it is only for a few selected people. Actually, the truth is that almost everyone can go on a water and/or dry fast. The only exception to this would be if you are suffering from a certain physical illness that would prevent you from fasting. I am not a medical expert, so I would suggest that you consult with your trusted physician before you engage in a real fasting experience. Still, it should be noted that fasting is a powerful way to heal the body. But, depending on the specific illness that you might have, it might not be safe for you. Again, just to be safe, it is best to ask your physician before you engage in the fasting experience. But, for most people, fasting is very safe and very healthy to do.

Once you verify that it is safe for you to go on a fast, you might still feel that it is too much for you. Many people think that they would not last even for a day without eating solid food. However, it should be clarified that a normal human body can safely last for days without food. Hence, you can fast, but it is up to you to do it and to finish it.

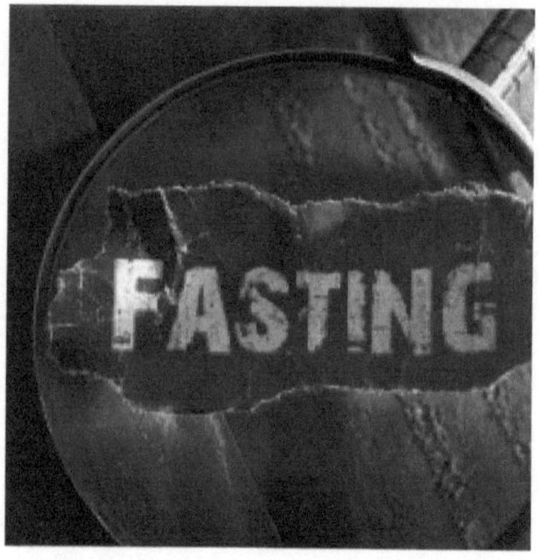

By the time that you finish reading this book, you will be equipped with the right knowledge about going on a real water and dry fast. If you really want to enjoy the many benefits of fasting, then I suggest that you do it immediately. After all, the only way for you to understand what fasting is and experience its enormous health and spiritual benefits is through actual practice.

The First Steps

The first step is to know whether you can go on a fast safely. Again, I would leave this to your physician since there can be lots of complicated matters in terms of health. The next step is to make a firm decision that you are finally going to do it—that yes, you are going to fast. Again, if you are just starting out, it is good to learn water fasting first before trying a dry fast. Going on a dry fast is optional. I know many spiritual seekers and health enthusiasts who are already happy and satisfied with water fasting. Although I have tried dry fasting so many times, I personally prefer going on a water fast.

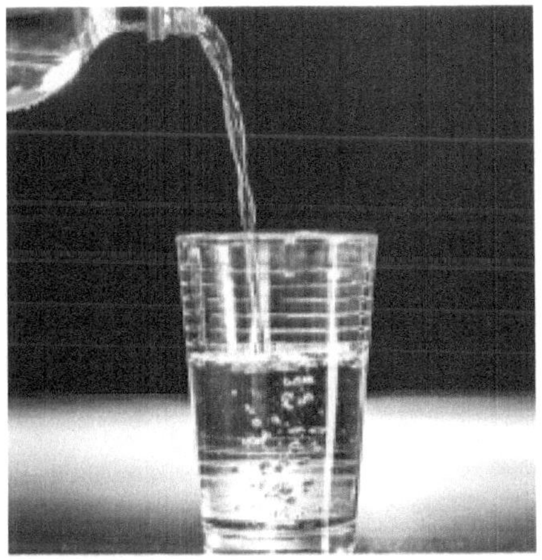

You do not need to go on a water fast for one whole day completely. For starters, you can gently ease in and prepare yourself by learning to fast little by little. For example, you can start out by skipping a meal, preferably dinner. Just get used to it for a few days. You can drink water when you feel hungry. Here is a pro tip: drink lots of water even *before* you feel hungry.

Once you can skip a meal, then you can take it a step further by skipping two meals. And, before you know it, you will get used to it and be able to easily go on a fast for a whole day. If you are daring enough, you can do it just the way I did it: just go on a 24-hour fast right away—starting right now.

Are You Feeling Tempted to Break the Fast?

When you go on a fast, it is very easy to be tempted to break it. This is something that many beginners often commit. You should overcome this temptation as much as possible. However, if it is too much for you, and if you fail by breaking the fast too quickly, do not be too hard on yourself.

To overcome this temptation, you should develop a stronger and more positive mindset. The real enemy here lies in the mind. By learning to deal with this enemy, you can overcome it and succeed in your fasting objective. But how exactly do you overcome this temptation to break the fast?

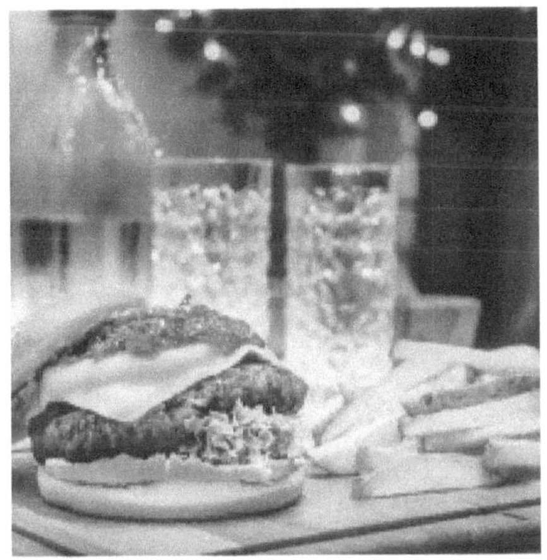

This strong temptation usually happens when you feel hungry. When this occurs, you may suddenly lose all willpower and simply give up. Even before you go on a fast, you should already expect for this to happen, so that you will be more prepared to face it when it finally comes.

A suggested way to get through this normal temptation is to drink more water. Another thing that you can do is simply to sleep on it. A common mistake is to spend so much time thinking about the temptation. You must realize that there is no way out of it except only to submit to it. However, submitting to this temptation would mean giving up your fast, which should not be an option unless only for compelling reasons.

Instead of dealing with the temptation by desperately trying to overcome it, you should simply overcome it by not paying any attention to it. If you can, get yourself busy with something else. A very common mistake is to continue to entertain the temptation in your mind. If you do this, the temptation will only get stronger and stronger, and this would not be beneficial for you. So, the proper approach is to ignore the temptation by focusing your mind on something else.

In any case, or if all efforts fail, there is no last resort but simply to overcome any and all temptations through the use of your pure willpower. This may be quite hard in the beginning, but you just have to give your body enough time to adjust to it. Soon enough, fasting for a day or even for two days would be very easy for you, and it would even be a very enjoyable experience.

Treat Yourself

You are not expected to be in a fasting state forever. There is a time to fast and a time to feast. When I was a beginner, I would eat all that I wanted to eat and really treat myself before going on a fast. I would usually fast for one to three days, sometimes longer. Feel free to treat yourself for a nice meal every now and then, especially before going on a fast—and remember that very full feeling.

Once we become full, we usually tend to not like the feeling of being too full, especially once you have gotten used to the fasting state. This is one of the reasons why we treat ourselves every now and then. It is not only to enjoy a delicious meal (including an unhealthy meal), but it is also to teach us how it feels to be too full. It usually gives a feeling that you do not want to eat again and that you may even miss the clean feeling of having an empty stomach.

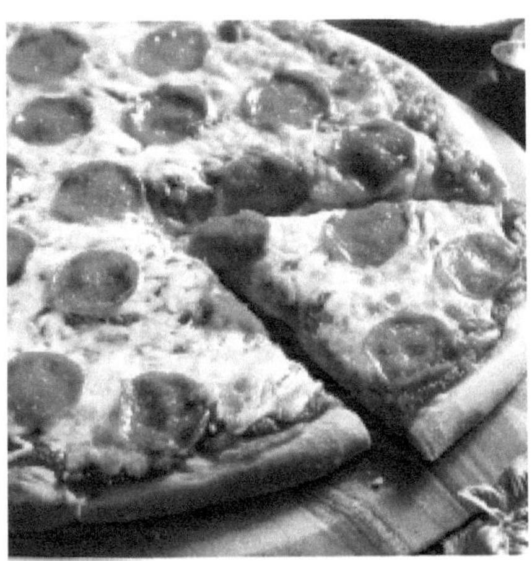

As much as possible, you should treat yourself to some healthy foods; but every now and then, it is not really prohibited to indulge in some unhealthy snacks. This is another benefit of fasting: You are no longer afraid to eat even unhealthy food because you know that your body has now become a powerful cleansing and healing machine. However, this does not mean that you must indulge in so much unhealthy foods. You should still avoid them as much as possible, but do not be afraid to treat yourself to some ice cream, chocolates, and pizza from time to time. After all, you deserve to be happy.

One-Day Fast

Now that you have more ideas about fasting, you can now challenge yourself for a real one-day fast. This is where you are going to fast for one whole day. I prefer to do it from waking up in the morning up to the next morning, or from one sunrise to the next.

There is usually no problem with fasting in the morning. A glass of water usually does the trick. This is true, especially if you have eaten a lot the night before. However, after a few hours, you may start to feel hungry. This is also usually the part where temptations will begin to creep in, telling you to break the fast already and just start over again some other time. However, if you do not get past this simple challenge, then you would never be able to complete a one-day fast. Therefore, be strong as much as you can. This is also the time when you need to exercise your willpower—and that is to stay true to the objective of completing a whole-day fast. Do not worry; remember that you will only be fasting for a day, so you should not be too hard on yourself. You can eat whatever you want after you fast. But, for now, you should stay strong and get through the phases of fasting in order to reap its wonderful benefits.

This is also a good time to remember the feeling of getting too full, especially after eating an unhealthy meal. Use your mind to discourage yourself from taking a bite of something, instead of allowing temptations to weaken your willpower.

You may face various challenges throughout the day, and even more so at night. You just have to stay strong. If it helps, read more books and watch videos about fasting during this time to help motivate you to complete your objective.

You might be surprised with how good your mind can be at convincing you to break the fast; but, do not listen to it. This is no longer about the mind or the thoughts that you should be thinking, but it is just a matter of becoming still and staying strong until the next sunrise (the time to break the fast). If you stay strong right now, you will surely be happy about it later. But, if you break the fast, you might just be disappointed as you just return to where you have always been. Think about it. Stay strong.

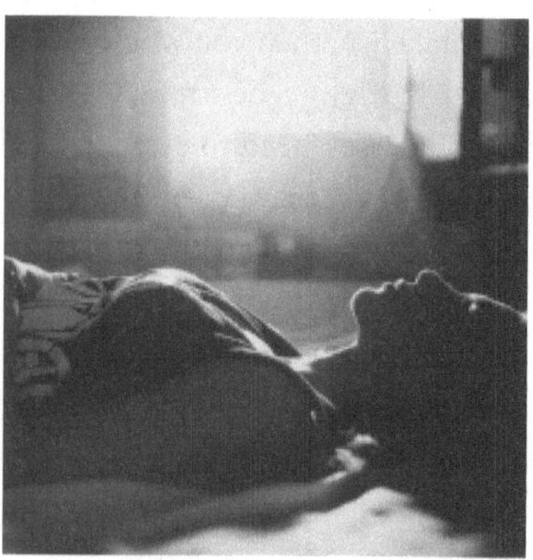

At any time during the day or night that you find it challenging, just lay in bed and relax. Just allow the time to pass. You do not need to do anything. You are already fasting right now—this is it, the one that you have been wondering about. The more that you stay in this zone, the more that your body is going to heal. Just relax, be still, and let go.

In the evening, if possible, sleep as early as you can. By the time you wake up, the Sun would be up, and you could finally congratulate yourself by breaking the fast—hence, it is called *breakfast*.

How to Break the Fast

Breaking the fast feels like a celebration, but you should break the fast gently; otherwise, you may suffer some stomach problems. You do not want to shock your digestive system and even your whole body with a sudden rush of food.

The proper way to break a fast is by eating a very light meal, such as fruits or vegetables. Drinking fresh fruit juice is also good. In any case, never break a fast with a heavy meal. You should ease into it slowly and gently. Gradually increase the amount of food little by little. This is also a good time to correct your eating habits if ever you started the fast with a very unhealthy diet.

You have probably heard about some Muslims who get rushed into the hospital during the Ramadan. Ramadan is a holy period of fasting for Muslims. If you do not break the fast gently, it can be bad for your body. There are really no strict rules on how to go about doing it, except only to do it gently with a very light meal and/or drink.

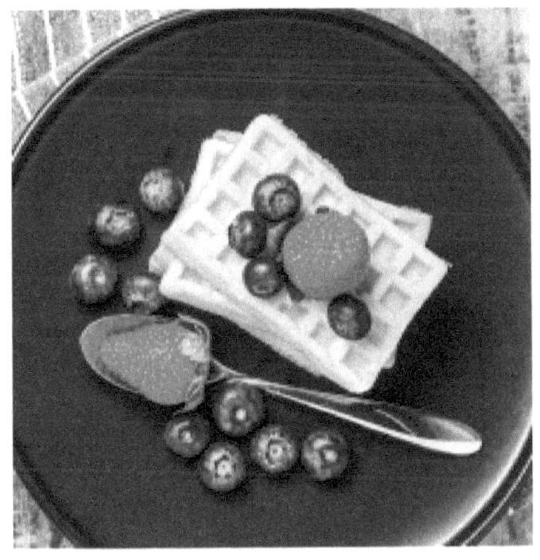

Breaking a fast is actually very simple and easy. It is good to start with something soft like vegetables. However, if this is not possible, just eat something that is very light. I remember a time when the only food I had to break the fast was chicken. So, I ate just about two bites of it. I also made sure to chew it well in my mouth so that my digestive system would not be surprised by the new load of food to digest. Still, it is strongly suggested to break a fast with something healthy, such as vegetables and fruits. I prefer sticking to vegetables and fruits since that is how I usually break my fast. Nevertheless, you have a choice on how you want to do it as long as you do it gently and slowly.

It should be clarified that in breaking a fast, do not just eat something that is healthy, but you should also eat lightly. This means that you should only eat a small quantity. In my case, for example, I would eat only a piece of banana or a few slices of apple. You should warm up your digestive system gradually. This is the right way to break a fast.

On Drinking Tea & Coffee

There are those who go on a fast wondering if it is still considered fasting if they drink coffee and/or tea during the fast. Technically speaking, it would no longer be called a water fast nor a dry fast if you drink tea or coffee during the fast. Therefore, if you really want to experience the full benefits of fasting, then you should avoid drinking tea or coffee during the fasting state.

However, there is also what is called the *liquid fast*. Liquid fasting, as the name already suggests, is where you only consume liquids during the fasting period. This is also a form of fasting that is lighter and easier than a water fast. Some people who want to go on a water fast also begin with a liquid fast.

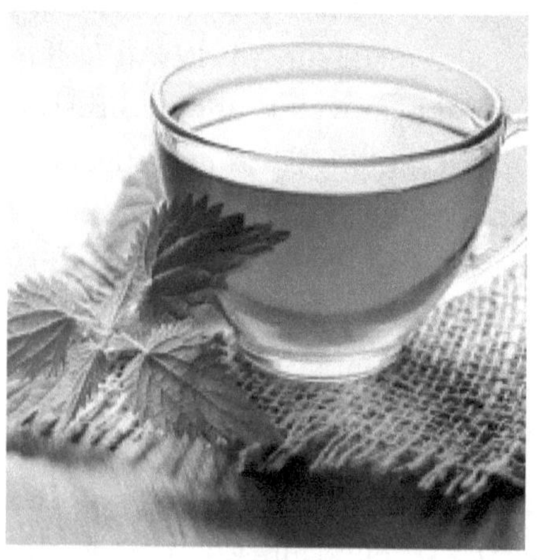

If you go on a liquid fast, you can drink coffee, milk, fresh fruit juice, tea, and even a hot cup of caramel or chocolate drink, among others. I also love liquid fasting, and I still practice it quite often to this day. However, it is less powerful than water fasting. But, it should be noted that liquid fasting is also a powerful healing technique, and that it has been practiced since ancient times.

Therefore, if you want to be able to drink tea and/or coffee during a fast, then you should do a liquid fast. When you are doing a liquid fasting, you should, as much as possible, drink only healthy beverages. However, I do know some people who also drink soda during this period. Although it may seem alright; but if you really want to get the powerful healing benefits of liquid fasting, you should stick to healthy beverages only. Therefore, stay away from sodas, beers, artificial beverages, and alcoholic beverages, among others. Stay liquid with natural drinks; stay clean.

Fasting for More than a Day

After being able to fast for a day, you can easily and gradually shift to fasting for two or three days. After that, you could easily fast for more than three days.

Indeed, a person in normal health can go on a fast safely for days. In fact, Moses and Jesus fasted for 40 days, as well as many other prophets and spiritual seekers.

In the beginning, it may be difficult to fast for three consecutive days. This is because the body has not yet adjusted to the fasted state, and your mind is not yet that confident to be able to do it.

Another thing that is important is to appreciate the beauty of the fasting state. During the very state when your stomach is empty and the body does not draw any energy from food but uses what remains of it as its energy primarily from excess calories and fats. The clean feeling that you have when you are fasting, as well as the clarity of mind and peacefulness of being—these are priceless.

If you are going on a fast for a longer period (more than a day), you should listen to your body. Take note that fasting should promote good health. I know someone who suddenly fasted for 48 hours. She was already shaking before she reached the 48th hour. This is the wrong way to do fasting. When the body already gives clear signals of discomfort, you should gently break the fast, and just try to fast again next time. Do not push your body beyond its current limits. Take note that fasting should be done gently and naturally.

Although it is normal and expected to experience some discomfort like a mild headache, a bit of stomach pain when hungry, and so on, you should listen to your body. When it sends you signals that are already alarming like a terrible headache or a trembling body, then you should break the fast. Many times, the body is simply shocked by the cleanliness of the fast. The woman I have mentioned, on the first try, her body ended up trembling; but on her second attempt to fast, her body was perfectly normal. It appears that her body just needed to adjust for some time. You need to give both your body and mind to adjust to the way of fasting. So, be patient and just enjoy the fast and all the benefits that fasting offers.

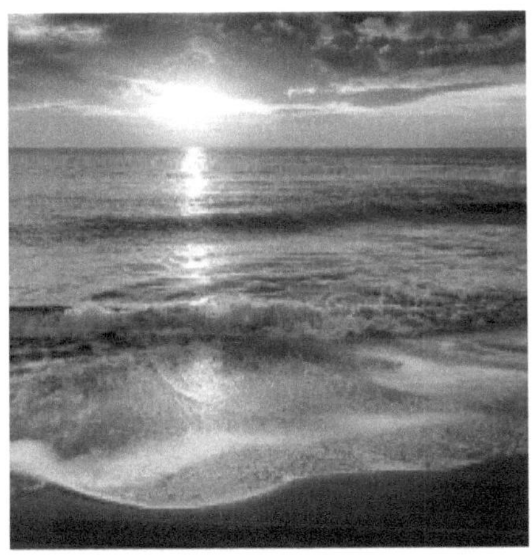

Instead of going on a long fast, you might also consider fasting every other day. I used to do this a few years ago. For example, I fasted on a Sunday, ate on Monday, then fasted again on Tuesday, ate on Wednesday, fasted on Thursday, and so on. It is simply fasting on alternate days of the week. You might want to try it and see how it works for you. During the days when you eat, make sure to charge your body with healthy food in order to be ready for the next day's fast.

If you intend to fast for a longer period, such as for a week or longer, know that the body will adjust. You will soon come into a point where you will no longer feel hungry at all. You will also experience the so-called *fasting high*. This is a state of mind that is very pleasant and wonderful. It may come and go, but you will most likely be able to experience it. It is also one of the reasons why some people engage in fasting.

The more that you fast, the more that your body will adjust, and the more that you will get used to it. However, as you undergo this stage, you must also be careful with how you are living your life. Be sure to move away from all stress and negative thoughts. As much as possible, only fill your mind with positive thoughts.

If you are just starting out, just aim to be able to fast for a day, and then two to three days. From here, it will be easy for you to make more adjustments, including extending your fasting days. It just really takes some time before the body can adjust to the fasting state, but it is nevertheless doable—and you can surely do it.

Meditation

If you are going on a fast, it is good to include the practice of meditation. You can also meditate whenever you feel like you are having a hard time during the fasting state. Meditation will help to clear your mind, as well as give you a deep sense of peace, which is quite rare judging by modern standards. In our modern world, the minds of the people are often bombarded with so many pressures and lots of stress. The minds of the people are often chaotic.

Regular practice of meditation has also been proven by conventional science to be beneficial for the body, as well as for mental health.

Contrary to what many people think, meditation is actually very easy to do. In fact, it is more about doing less than requiring you to do something more. It is about being still and relaxed. The truth is that everyone can meditate, but the question is if you would once you learn how to do it. The most common reason why people do not meditate is because they are busy. If you really want to make any progress in meditation, then you must make time for it. The modern world will always give you lots of things to do and worry about, and it is up to you to finally make the decision and make the time to spend in meditation.

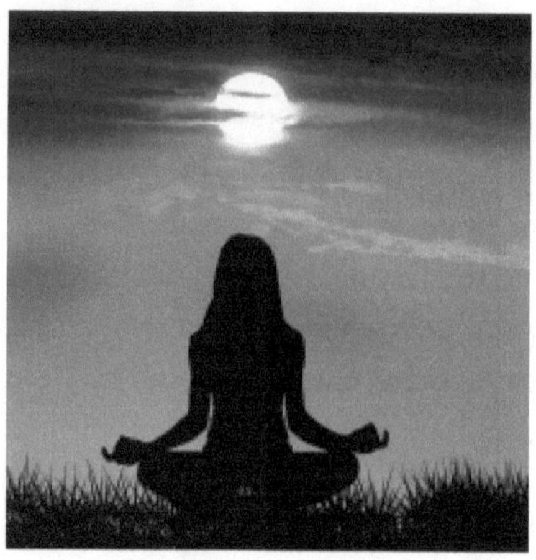

Meditation has been practiced for many centuries. How meaningful it is would depend on how much meaning that you give to it. Nevertheless, it should be noted that meditation is, first and foremost, a spiritual practice.

There are many ways to meditate, but you do not really need to learn all of them. Having said that, here is a powerful and simple meditation technique that you can do:

Be comfortable and relax. You can meditate in any position that you want. Close your eyes, and do not think about anything. Breathe and let go. Now, begin to say the following mantra: *Lord Jesus Christ, Son of God, have mercy on me.*" The said mantra is also known as *The Jesus Prayer*. It has been used by various monks and spiritual seekers for so many years. You can use the said mantra even if you are not a follower of Christ. It is good to use this mantra because it has already been charged with divine energy for a very long time. By using this mantra, you get to partake in the powerful divine energy that the mantra is charged with.

Say your mantra gently, lovingly, and repeatedly. As you are saying the mantra, gently focus on it. Do not imagine anything, and do not think about anything. Nothing must exist in the mind but the mantra. If thoughts continue to arise in the mind, and this is something that is very common, simply ignore them. Only focus on the mantra. Nothing must exist in the mind but the mantra. Let go of everything else.

Meditate for as long as you like. The more that you meditate, the more that you will be able to access a deeper state of mind and being. At any time that you want to end this meditation, simply bring your awareness back to your body, slowly move your fingers and toes, and very gently open your eyes.

It is recommended to practice the said meditation at least twice daily. If you can meditate more, then do so. The more that you meditate, the more that you will improve and reach deeper states of consciousness. Regular practice of the said meditation will also give you a profound calmness and stillness, as well as peace of mind.

How to Handle Mood Swings

People who are not used to fasting usually have a hard time managing their temper. In this regard, the practice of meditation will also be very helpful as it can quickly give you peace of mind. However, there are other measures that you can take to resolve this issue.

If you know that you are one of the many who have a hard time managing their moods, you should, as much as possible, stay away from people during the fasting period as you will most likely not be one of the nicest people to have around. Do not worry, this is just in the beginning; as your body adjusts and gets used to the fasting state, the more that you will be able to manage those mood swings.

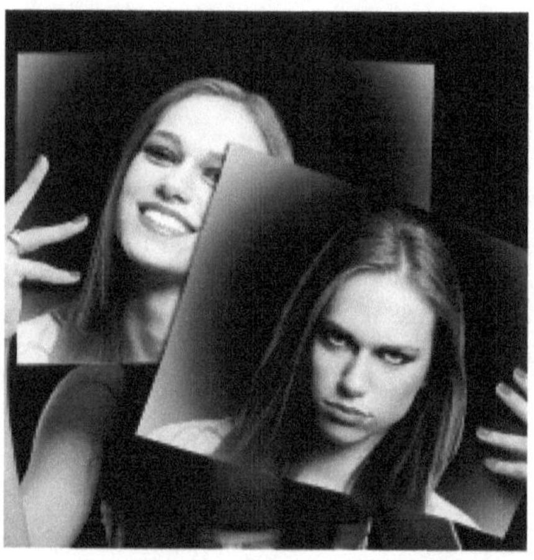

Another thing that you can do is to drink more water. The mood swings usually occur because of hunger. By drinking lots of water, hunger will decrease. This will give you enough space to deal with the undesirable mood.

If you are the spiritual type, praying also helps. It is worth noting that many prophets and spiritual masters also fasted. In fact, even Jesus Christ also fasted.

Last but not least, you just have to overcome it using your willpower. The practice of fasting is also an effective way to develop one's willpower. If you can overcome the challenge of something so basic (important) as the appetite, then there are so many things in the world that you can also overcome.

The Wonders of Autophagy

Autophagy means *self-eating*. When the body goes into a state of fasting and runs out of energy reserve, it will soon start consuming the bad cells in the body. Autophagy was discovered by the Japanese scientist named Yoshinori Ohsumi, for which he was awarded the Nobel Prize.

This process of autophagy is a very powerful healing process. It may be quite uncomfortable as you are fasting, but it is only a sign that your body is healing. Many times, the healing power of the body is prevented because so much energy is used for digesting food. But, when you fast, the body can utilize its powerful healing force optimally. Indeed, so many diseases can be cured and also prevented when you allow the body to undergo autophagy every now and then—and this is one of the benefits of fasting.

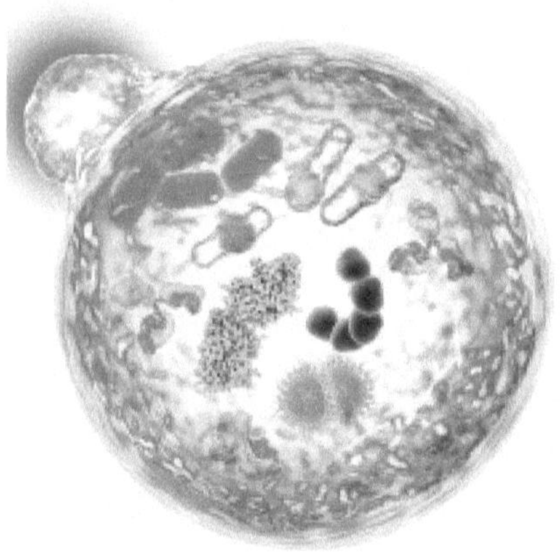

If you want to do fasting for healing, then this is the way to go. Whether you do water fasting or dry fasting, it will all lead you to this powerful state of healing.

Take note that the body must first use its default energy reserve before you can reach the state of autophagy. There is no specific length of time on when you will reach this state. If you have taken a heavy meal prior to the fast, then you may need more time before you can reach autophagy. On average, you will reach autophagy in about a 24-hour timeline. If you can fast for a longer period, then you will reach a more powerful state of autophagy. As you can see, the longer that you can fast, the more that your body will heal.

On Dry Fasting

Once you get used to water fasting, you can easily switch to dry fasting. Dry fasting is where you totally give up consuming food and drinks, including water. There are people who claim that they could do this for a very long period, even for several months. However, it should be noted that it is not completely safe. In fact, some of the followers of that movement have died due to the practice they were doing.

Still, it is worth noting that dry fasting is also a powerful fast. In fact, it is said that it is even more powerful than water fasting. Personally, I am already happy with water fasting. I have tried dry fasting many times, and I also liked it but it is not something that I would recommend doing for a long time. Once again, listen to your body.

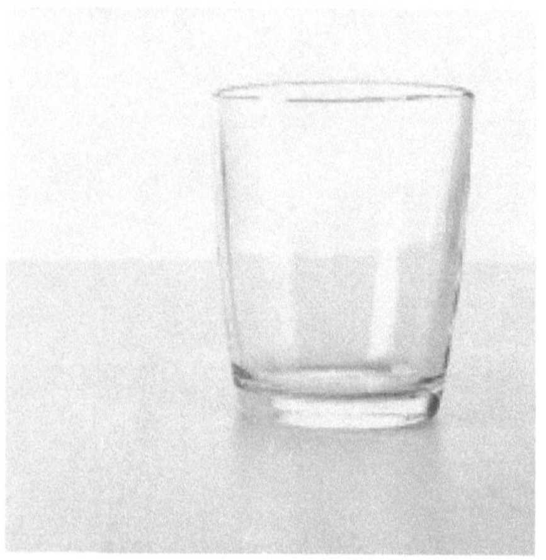

Shifting into a dry fast is very easy once you can already do a water fast. In fact, I did not have a hard time at all. It may just sound scary or difficult, but it actually is not. But, before you go on a dry fast, be sure to accomplish water fasting first. This is because once you can already do water fasting, then dry fasting would also be easy for you.

Breathe

Many people do not breathe properly, while many others do not breathe as much. When was the last time that you took a real deep breath?

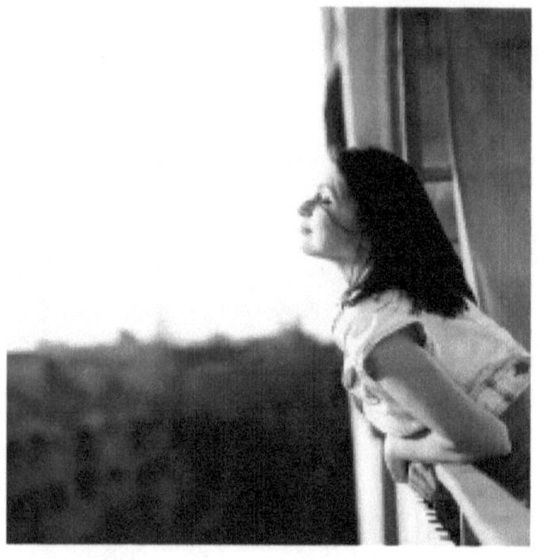

Breathing is good. The breath is also commonly used in meditation. Breath is life. Here is an exercise that you can do:

Assume a comfortable position and relax. Breathe gently through your nose. Gently focus on your breathing. Many times, we take our breaths for granted, failing to realize that a simple break in this cycle of inhalation and exhalation would mean death. This time, be aware of your breath. If thoughts arise in the mind, ignore them. Only focus on the breath. This is also known as *breathing meditation*. Breathe, relax, and let go.

When you are fasting, and you feel like having a hard time, do this exercise and see how you feel afterward. Remember that he who meditates on the breath actually meditates on life. Breath is life.

35

Fasting is Simple

Fasting is very simple. In fact, it is more about not doing anything rather than having to do something. Whether you go on a water fast or a dry fast, it is all about relaxing and becoming still. This is its big difference from the modern world that always pressures us to do something. Fasting is a state of deep relaxation and peace. You may not yet appreciate this if you are a beginner, but once you get used to it and taste the beauty of fasting, you will definitely understand what this is all about.

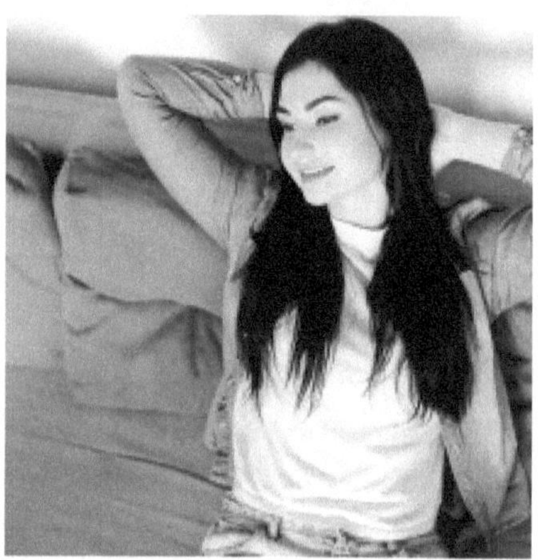

Now is the time for you to relax from all the pressures of the day and stresses of life. Do not try to complicate fasting. It is when you make it complicated that makes it difficult.

Our ancestors also fasted since there were times when food was scarce. Even today, it is not uncommon for tribal people to naturally engage in a fast because of their environment. It is the environment of the modern world that you should be cautious of since we are bombarded with lots of unhealthy foods and drinks, as well as vices.

So, if you want to go on a fast, just do it. How do you do it? Do nothing (stop eating). It is that simple. Can you do this simple thing for me, please? It is for your own good.

Stop Thinking

There is an ancient saying that goes like this: If you have already decided and your body can do it, then just do it without ever thinking while you are doing it.

Many times, it is our own mind that prevents us from doing something good. It is also not uncommon for those who are wanting to fast to fail because of too much thinking.

It is already expected that you will experience some discomfort when you fast, especially if you are a beginner. Therefore, when this happens, do not be discouraged because getting hungry is a normal part of fasting. In fact, if you do not want to get hungry, then do not fast.

But, just to make you feel better, know that it is actually when you are hungry that you are fasting. Hunger is the sign that you are finally doing it right.

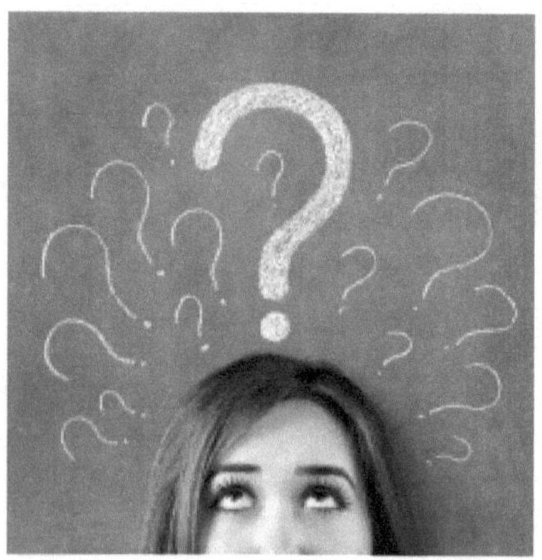

You can expect that your thoughts will start to play around and will soon discourage you from staying in a fasting state. Do not listen to those negative thoughts. If possible, just sleep through it. Soon enough, you will surely thank yourself for not submitting to those weak and negative thoughts.

Therefore, the next time you feel hungry while fasting, congratulate yourself instead of thinking of ways to run away from fasting. It only means that you are doing the right thing, and you are doing a very good thing.

What if I Fail?

Except when the body is sending you a signal that you should break the fast, then there is no reason for you to allow yourself to fail. If it is the body that wants you to stop the fast, then it is not a failure, but it is a natural part of the life of fasting. But, if it is just your mind that you are submitting to, specifically the negative and discouraging thoughts, then do your best to overcome them.

But, okay, what if you fail? If it would make you feel any better, I was actually a big failure when it comes to fasting. It probably took me more than five attempts before I managed to do a simple 24-hour fast. I would usually fail somewhere in the middle of fasting.

If ever you also fail and submit to your weaknesses, learn from the experience. Do not be too hard on yourself, but do not be too kind on yourself either; otherwise, you might never be able to succeed at any attempt at fasting. So, learn from the experience, and reflect on what made you submit to your weaknesses.

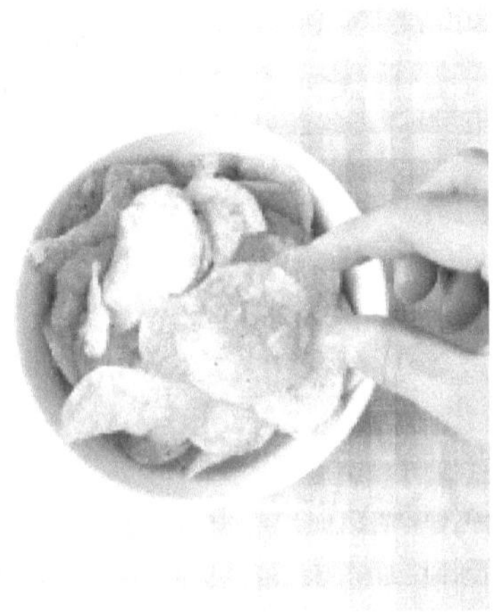

Take note of every wrong thought that you have failed to overcome, so that you will be more ready to face them the next time you fast. There is a very high chance that you will be facing the same thoughts again soon, so be more prepared. You will keep facing these challenges until you rise above them.

As you can see, there is so much that you can learn from fasting, and it will also develop your character. Even if you fall, just stand and try again. If you do not give up, you will never lose.

Grounding & Centering Exercise

Before you decide to end your fast and submit to your weakness, it might help to do the following exercise first. This exercise, which is known as the *Tree Exercise*, will keep you grounded and help you find your center. It can also help to keep you strong when you are already feeling discouraged. Here are the steps:

Stand with your feet touching the ground. It is ideal to do this with your bare feet touching the fresh soil of the Earth. However, if this is not possible, you can still do this even while wearing shoes and even if you are in the office or in your room. The important thing is to keep your feet flat on the floor.

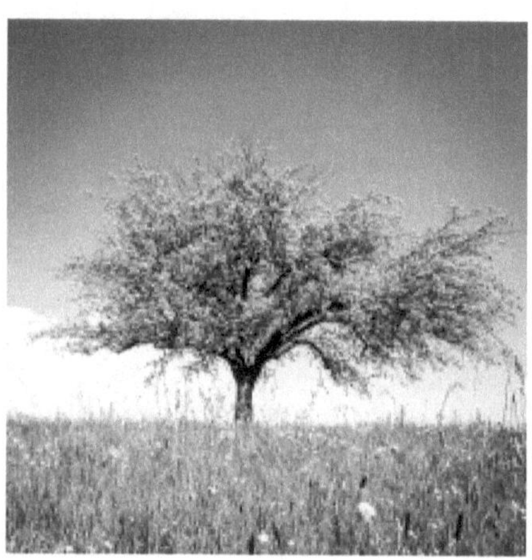

Now, imagine roots like those of a tree slowly coming out from the soles of your feet. Gently send your roots down into the Earth. Send them as far as they want to go until they stop naturally.

Feel and appreciate the connection that you now have with the Earth. Know that Mother Earth is very much alive. Spend as much time as you want, feeling connected to the Earth.

Many times, this is already enough. But, if you want to take this exercise a step further, you can *drink* the fresh green energy of the Earth. By now, you must be hungry, so feel free to take as much of the Earth's energy as you want.

To do this, inhale—and as you inhale, see and feel that you are drinking the Earth's fresh green energy through your roots. Allow the energy to pass through your roots, and then through the soles of your feet, and into your body, thereby charging you with the Earth's pure and fresh green energy. Continue this until your whole body is fully recharged.

At any time that you want to end this exercise, thank Mother Earth, and then imagine your roots slowly fading away.

This is a powerful exercise that is also used in some spiritual circles. The more that you practice it, the more powerful its effects are going to be.

You might be wondering, is this all just a trick of the mind? Well, perhaps. But, just so you know, there are many spiritual people who believe that what you imagined actually happened in another dimension. So, yes, it is more than a trick of the mind because it is real.

Nevertheless, whether real or not, there is a good chance that you will benefit from this exercise. You will be able to feel more grounded, recharged, and also find your center. Just give it a try and see how it works for you.

Fasting State vs. Full State

It is also a recommended practice to compare your feeling between the fasting state and when you are very full with food. You may soon start to appreciate the beautiful and clean feeling of being on a fast.

Of course, I know the feeling of being full, especially after eating my favorite dish. However, after I came to know fasting better, I also started to look for it: That feeling of being empty and clean. It is unlike anything. You also know that your whole body is healing at all levels, which is a really good plus. Not only that, but you also know that fasting is a very effective way to lose weight. In fact, when it comes to losing weight, I strongly recommend fasting. Do not mind those who say that you will only be losing water weight. The people who say that are only those who have not yet discovered the wonders that only fasting can bring.

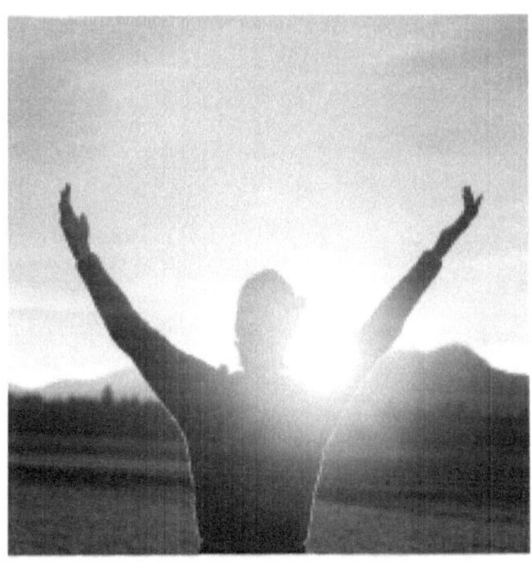

The important thing here is to appreciate the feeling when you are fasting. If you cannot appreciate that, it might be difficult for you to really love fasting. But, once you fall in love with fasting, it will be much easier to do because you will be able to do it with passion, and you know that it is something that you want. Once you develop this strong will to fast, then fasting will become significantly easier for you.

When your tummy is full of food, it does bring pleasure—but it is only a short moment of pleasure. This is unlike the state of fasting where you can keep it for as long as you want, until you finally break it. But then again, you can always return to it at any time you want.

Another thing that I love about fasting is the feeling when I wake up in the morning. I feel very clean inside. And, if I ever decide to break the fast, breakfast becomes a really meaningful one.

Keep a Journal

Although not necessary, you might also want to keep a journal. I know many people who fast who say that their journal has been really helpful to them on their fasting journey. You can give it a try and see how it works for you.

Keeping a fasting journal is easy. You can have your journal in a notebook just like the traditional way, but you can also take advantage of technology. In this case, you can keep your journal by having a file on your computer or even on your smartphone. There are now many applications that you can download that will allow you to keep some notes and entries.

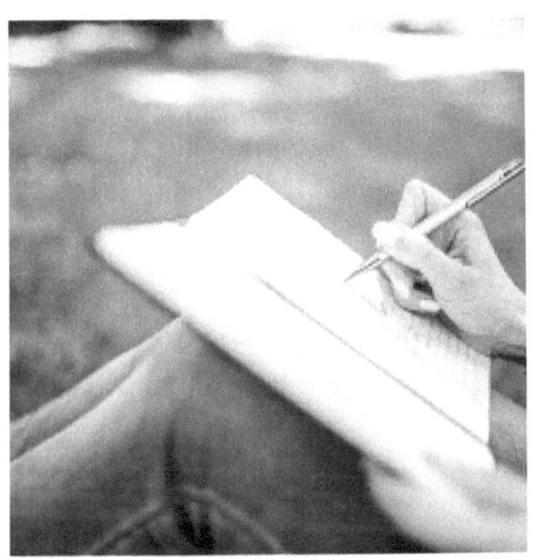

So what should you write in your journal? You are free to write everything that you want in your journal that is related to fasting. Some suggested ideas would be the reasons why you want to go on a fast, the negative and discouraging thoughts that you still find difficult to overcome, your fasting objectives, and the thoughts and emotions that you are having, among others.

In the beginning, you might not yet appreciate the value of journaling. The value of a journal appreciates over time. So, just keep writing and recording, and you will soon thank yourself for doing it.

When you write your fasting journal, you should remember to always be open and honest with yourself. There are some people who commit the mistake of only acknowledging their strengths and keeping a blind eye on their weaknesses. Take note that the more weaknesses that you are able to identify and write in your journal, the more beneficial it will be for you because it will allow you to better understand the things that you have to work on.

Journalling will also allow you not only to have a clear record of your experiences but also to be able to view yourself from a different perspective—from a view that is unbiased and clear.

If ever you come to love the art of journaling, you might want to journal about your life and many other things other than fasting. It is said that journaling is also an effective way to destress and find more meaning in life.

Stay Motivated

The fasting journey can be challenging. But, it is up to you how you will manage the challenges along the way to fasting greatness. It is important to keep yourself motivated. Many times, those who fast are only motivated in the beginning, but then they fall away from the path at the very first feeling of hunger.

Indeed, a strong willpower is essential to succeed at fasting. When it comes to having a strong willpower, your motivation is important. You should keep yourself motivated not only at the start of the fast, but also during the whole stretch of the fast itself.

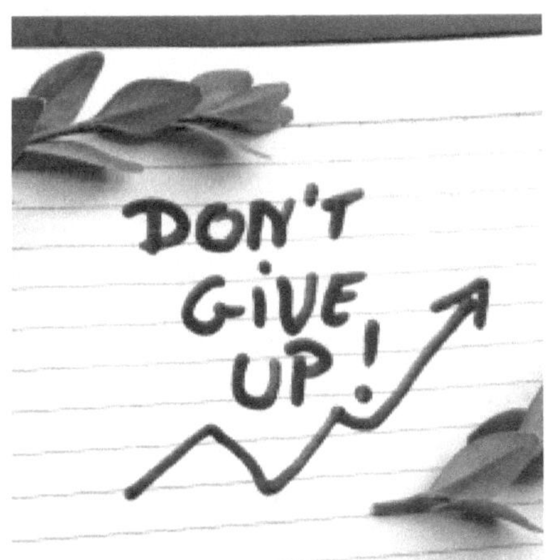

But how can you keep yourself motivated for the duration of the fast? Well, there are some tricks and tips that you can do. One of the best ways to keep your motivation strong and elevated is to read more about the benefits of fasting, as well as to watch videos on fasting. This is also a good way to remind yourself why you are doing it.

Another thing that you can do is to fast with a friend. This way, you would not have to face the challenges alone. However, in choosing a friend to do fasting with, be sure to choose someone who is also serious about fasting. If the person would only discourage you along the way and be the first one to give up, then it would be better for you to just fast on your own. It is suggested that you choose someone who has already successfully done a fast. This way, you know that you are working with someone who could actually do it, and you might also learn from them.

When it comes to being motivated, now is probably the best time to consult your journal. Read and see your fasting progress. Be sure to review the reasons that you have for fasting, so that you can remind yourself of the importance of fasting in your life.

If possible, you can also attend workshops on fasting. From time to time, yoga and other spiritual centers give workshops that are related to fasting.

Sometimes, your motivation may just disappear for some time. During these moments, it is up to you alone to just be strong and go through the challenges. Do not worry; you can do it. After all, there is nothing that you need to do. You just have to be still, relax, and let go. You can definitely do this.

Sleep

The fasting state has a lot to do with the passage of time. When fasting, and to actually make it, sometimes the best advice is simply to sleep through it. I am not saying that you should spend your whole time in bed; but when things get tough for you, it is advisable to just relax in bed—and if you can, sleep. It is worth noting that it is still considered fasting even when you are asleep.

When you sleep, time passes significantly more quickly, and you will not have to go through the undesirable feeling of hunger and all the temptations that come with it.

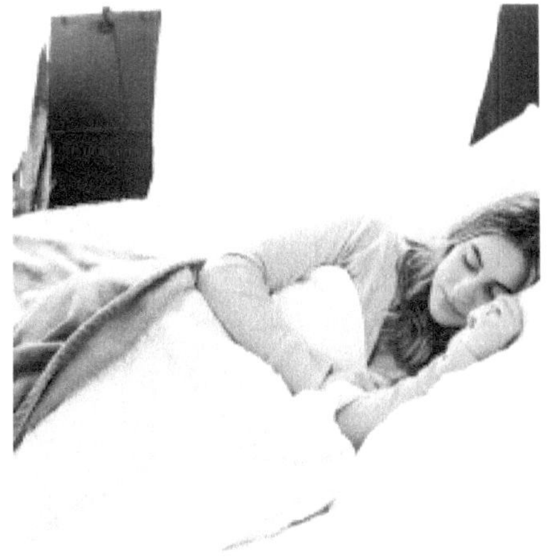

When lying in bed to sleep, be careful not to fall into the traps of negative thoughts. Many times, this is the part where you will start to wonder about finally giving up. Instead of thinking about these things that are counterproductive to your objective, do not think at all. Just relax your body and mind—and sleep.

If you cannot sleep, just rest your eyes and your body. Again, do not think about anything. If you will think, make sure that it is something pleasant or at least something that would encourage you to continue the fasting journey.

After you awake from the sleep/rest, you will have a much clearer mind to decide—and you will most likely be very happy that you have not yet broken your fast.

Add a Little Each Time

This advice is something that I learned from the stories of the Desert Father and Mothers of Egypt. They were the early Christian hermits and spiritual seekers who lived in the desert of Egypt.

If I remember it correctly, it is about a monk who was fasting and was already being tempted to break his fast. Instead of submitting to the temptation right away, he said that he will break the fast after three hours. When the said three hours came, he said that he will just wait for another three hours. He continued this process until he was soon able to complete his fasting period.

You do not need to be a desert monk to be able to do this. You can apply the same or similar technique when you are fasting. Instead of submitting to your weakness by breaking your fast, you can tell yourself, "Okay, after two hours." When the designated time lapses, repeat it again.

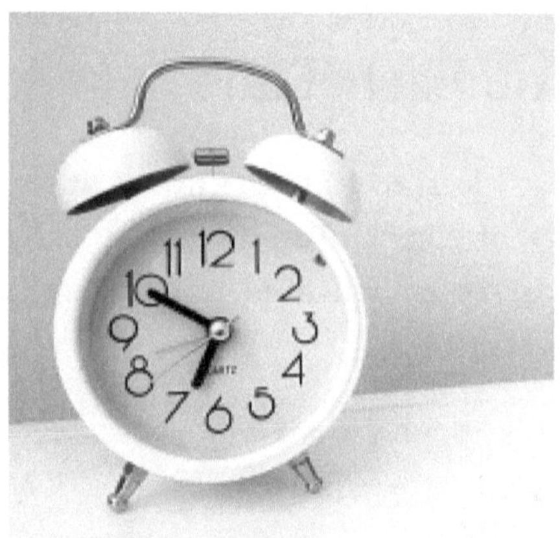

This is like the baby steps to fasting. Instead of immediately telling yourself to fast for 24 hours, try only for two or three hours. When the time lapses and you know that you can still do it, then give it another two hours until you finally complete the intended period for fasting.

Fasting as a Way of Life

Fasting can be made a way of life. This does not mean that you should fast forever, but you can easily incorporate fasting into your weekly schedule. For me, personally, I go on a fast after I indulge in a heavy meal.

Fasting will also encourage you to live a healthy lifestyle. The more that you fast, the healthier you are going to be.

Still, remember to listen to your body. If your body signals you to stop, then stop. After all, it is very easy to return to fasting at any time that you want. Do not be too hard on yourself. In fact, fasting is a way of loving yourself.

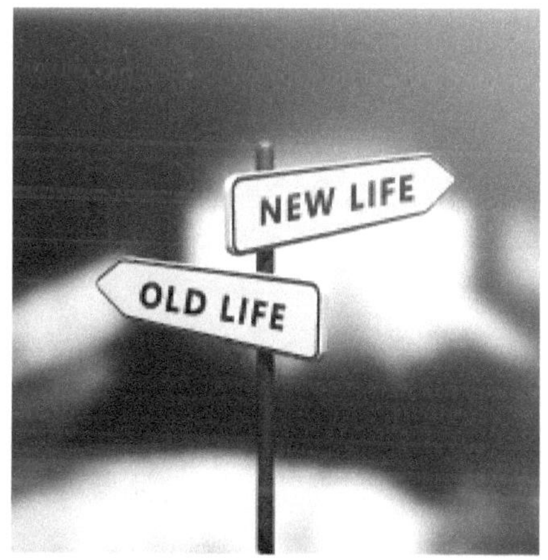

As you go through life's journey, you will meet various joys and challenges. Fasting will help you to be in touch with yourself. It cleanses not only the body, but also the mind. And, if you are also into spirituality like I am, then you will definitely find the fasting state so wonderful because it will allow you to be closer to your soul and to rely on God instead of your own strength.

Now that you have a good foundation on fasting, it is now up to you to get into the adventure and experience it yourself. I wish you all the best on your fasting journey!

A Sacred Call

I hope that you have enjoyed reading this book. Our humble journey ends here. But, before I let you go, there is something that I want to share with you. I have been practicing Witch for more than 20 years; I have always been attuned to nature, and I am now a follower of Jesus Christ. It is interesting to know that many witches and wizards these days are also turning to Christ for genuine spirituality and for more magic.

Shortly after Christ was born, He was visited by the three magi, which some people these days refer to as the three wise men. Based on the original text, the word *magi* was used. The word *magi* is the plural of the word *magus*—and the word *magus* is where the word *magic* came from. Hence, Jesus was visited by three magical practitioners. The church does not want to talk about it and even tried to change the word into wise men or even the three kings, as if to hide its real meaning. But, indeed, three magical practitioners came after Jesus was born.

In my life, despite all the magic and rituals that I have learned, I came to a point of complete darkness and depression. My magic could not save me. That was the time when Jesus came and rescued me. I have been serving Him since then.

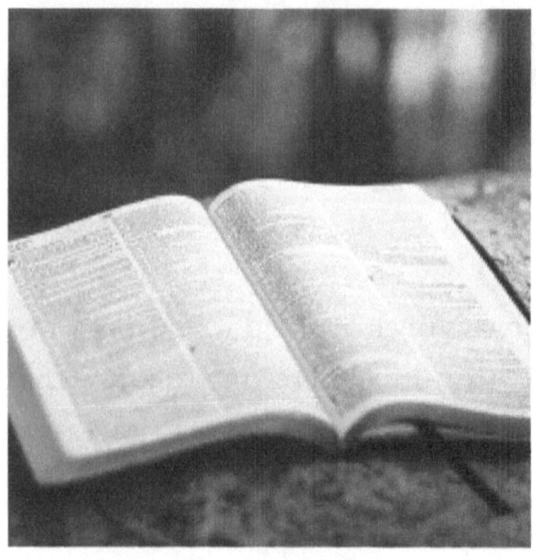

I would like to ask my dear reader to kindly give Christ a chance in your life. Forget about what you think you know about Him from what you have learned from religion and other people. You can start with a clean slate and get to know Him on your own. In this regard, I highly suggest starting out by reading the Bible. No, you do not need to read the whole Bible. You can easily start by reading the *Book of Matthew*, which also happens to be the first book in the New Testament of the Bible. This is a good way to know about the life and teachings of Jesus Christ. Do not worry, it is not a long book. In fact, I managed to finish reading it in just one sitting. Just please give it a try and see how it works for you.

Unlike other gods out there who do not care about you and would require a complicated ritual before they pay attention to you, Jesus is always with you, and He loves you. In fact, He loves you so much that He already suffered and died for you, so that you can enjoy salvation with Him in paradise.

The period of fasting is also a good time to work on your spiritual life. I sincerely hope that you may give Christ a chance. He might just change your life forever.

With light and love, Blessed Be!

Don't miss out!

Visit the website below and you can sign up to receive emails whenever Merryl Kowalska publishes a new book. There's no charge and no obligation.

https://books2read.com/r/B-A-OMZV-JDJEC

BOOKS 2 READ

Connecting independent readers to independent writers.

Did you love *Water Fasting & Dry Fasting for Beginners*? Then you should read *White Magic Manual*[1] by Merryl Kowalska!

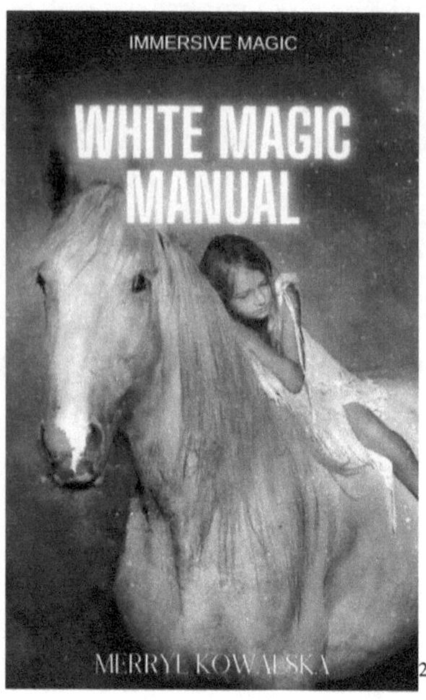

[2]

Immersive Magic: White Magic Manual is an occult manual that teaches the fine and sacred art of white magic. White magic has existed for centuries, and it is also an excellent practice for those who are starting out on their magical journey. Since you will be dealing with white magic, you can rest assured that you will only be dealing with good forces, and that the magic that you will cast will work for what is good. Hence, it is a very safe approach to the magical arts, and you will definitely learn a great deal from this practice.

---

1. https://books2read.com/u/4D6wAk

2. https://books2read.com/u/4D6wAk

Immersive Magic: White Magic Manual is written in an easy-to-understand format, so that you can focus more on learning the teachings and practicing the techniques. We will be discussing universal principles that apply to all forms of magic. Therefore, by learning about the art of white magic, you will also have a better understanding of all other magical art forms.

The good news is that white magic is not difficult to learn. In fact, it is one of the best ways to begin a magical journey. I personally know some practitioners of the craft who stick to learning and practicing white magic alone since they are already very happy and satisfied with it.

White magic is a complete magical system in and of itself. It also has many branches, just in case you want to specialize in a particular field of white magic later on. The white magic that we are going to discuss is completely based on universal laws and principles, so it will apply to whatever magical practice that you might be interested in.

Immersive Magic: White Magic Manual lays down the foundational teachings and practices of magic with a special relation to white magic. It should be noted as early as now that this book is not merely a manual of information, but it presents an invitation to a real magical journey.

Are you ready to take this journey -- a journey to a world of pure and divine magic? If yes, then let me now welcome you into this wonderful living universe of true magic paved into the ways of the right-hand path of magic -- behold the true power and manifestation of white magic.

Read more at https://www.czlibrary.com/.

Also by Merryl Kowalska

Immersive Magic
A Guide to Acquiring an Astral Magic Wand
Solitary Witchcraft for Beginners
Faerie Magick for Beginners
Magical Experiments That You Can Do at Home
Pendulum Dowsing Mastery Codex
White Magic Manual
Immersive Magic: Creating Energy Constructs
Beat Casino Games Using Psychic Techniques

Standalone
How to Be a Freelance Writer
Conjuration of the Demon Eryezel
Magical Cleansing and Defensive Techniques
Magick Black Book: Creating Magical Imbalances
The I Am of All Things and the None Self
Water Fasting & Dry Fasting for Beginners

Watch for more at https://www.czlibrary.com/.

www.ingramcontent.com/pod-product-compliance
Lightning Source LLC
Chambersburg PA
CBHW051814130726
47987CB00003B/1253